I0707830

16:8
Intermittent
Fasting

Dealing with Obesity
And Weight Loss

By

Dr. Betty G. Boice

Disclaimer!

Copyright © 2023 by Betty G. Boice

All rights reserved. No part of this publication may be reproduced, distributed, or transmitted in any form or by any means, including photocopying, recording, or other electronic or mechanical methods, without the prior written permission of the publisher, except in the case of brief quotations embodied in critical reviews and certain other noncommercial uses permitted by copyright law.

Table of Contents

About the author

Dr. Betty G. Boice, a distinguished expert in nutrition and wellness with a Ph.D. in Nutritional Sciences, is a trusted authority in the field of intermittent fasting. Her extensive research contributions, showcased in reputable journals and conferences, solidify her expertise. Driven by a commitment to evidence-based practices, she engages audiences through her accessible writing style in health publications, podcasts, and television programs. Dr. Boice's holistic approach aims to empower individuals in achieving health and fitness goals, as reflected in her comprehensive guide on intermittent fasting. Whether new to fasting or experienced, readers can benefit from her insights for a journey towards optimal health and well-being.

Introduction

Hey there, health explorer! Get ready to dive into the wild world of intermittent fasting with the one and only Dr. Betty G. Boice – your ticket to a healthier, happier you! Now, I know what you're thinking: fasting, really? Don't worry, we're not sending you on a hunger strike; we're just here to sprinkle a little science on your plate and make wellness way more exciting.

So, picture this: you, Dr. Boice, and a bunch of fascinating facts about how what you eat (and don't eat) can turn you into a health ninja. Forget the jargon and complicated stuff; we're breaking it down into bite-sized, chewable pieces – pun totally intended!

In the next few pages, we're going to uncover the mystery behind intermittent fasting. Spoiler alert: it's not rocket science (though Dr. Boice could probably explain that too). From the basics to the "aha!" moments, we're on a mission to make this whole fasting thing as easy as pie (without the guilt).

But who is Dr. Betty G. Boice, you ask? Oh, just your friendly neighborhood nutrition superhero with a Ph.D. in making science cool. She's been diving deep into the world of fasting, so you don't have to. And the best part? She's not here to tell you to eat kale all day (unless you want to, of course).

This isn't your average health lecture; it's more like having a chat with a witty friend who just happens to know a ton about making your body feel awesome. Dr. Boice will guide you through the sciencey stuff with a sprinkle of humor and a dash of enthusiasm, making this journey as enjoyable as a cheat day without the guilt trip.

So, grab your favorite snack (ironic, right?), kick back, and let's go on a hilarious and enlightening adventure into the world of intermittent fasting. Spoiler alert 2: It's going to be a game-changer, and you might just end up loving your body a little more. Ready? Let's roll!

Five Main Steps on the way to Start 16:8 Intermittent fasting and the way to not Fail in it at the very start

The 16:8 fasting is possibly the simplest weight-loss and wellness method you'll find. So, if you're reading this book, you're probably a beginner during this method, want to undertake it out, and see for yourself how it'll benefit, right? you'll also be doing it but want to urge a far better result. So, I'm here to offer you 5 main steps on the way to start 16:8 intermittent fasting and the way to not fail in it at the very start.

STEP NUMBER 1: Understand How 16:8 Works

OK, so for those that aren't sure what 16:8 really is, let me explain it a touch. Just to make sure we're on an equivalent page. 16:8 may be a sort of intermittent fasting once you eat during the 8 hour window. During these 8 hours, you'll eat all of your meals and snacks. and therefore the rest 16 hours you fast. During your fasting window, you'll only drink unsweetened drinks, like water, tea or coffee.

But why do you have to choose intermittent fasting?

Well, it's efficient thanks to reducing, improving blood glucose, boosting brain function and increasing longevity. Also, the 16:8 pattern is basically flexible and straightforward to follow because you opt for the foremost convenient timing of your eating and fasting windows.

For example, you'll eat between noon and eight PM, which suggests you will only go to fast overnight and skip breakfast. It's super beneficial to stay with this type over the future because without counting every single calorie, you are still losing weight. But as simple as it sounds, I do know that it is often complicated at the very beginning. So let's move to a different step.

STEP NUMBER 2: Fighting your hunger pangs.

You might be battling your hunger at the very beginning of 16:8. I'm not gonna lie: you'll get hungry!

It's just because your body doesn't want to go long periods without food.

Think of your stomach as something that must be trained. It means fasting is going to be difficult. But after a 3–5- day transition, your body will become easier without stuffing a lot of food into your stomach.

 I strongly suggest keeping yourself busy to remain on target,

especially at the very beginning. It's much easier to stay to your fast if you do not have plenty of time to snack. Because come on, guys, bored eating is bad eating!

STEP NUMBER 3: Drink a lot of water.

OK, so another MUST thing to try to do during 16:8 fasting: DRINK YOUR WATER! albeit you are not fasting, I'm pretty sure you are not drinking enough of it. Right? During fasting, it's really important to stay up your water intake. Water cleans out your whole system and effectively removes toxins from your body. beverages regularly can assist you reduce calorie intake because people often mistake thirst for hunger.

So here's the tip: drink a minimum of 8 glasses of water a day. confirm you drink a glass of water at the very first thing within the morning and before every meal. That's four glasses already! afterward, you'll notice that the beverage is popping into a habit.

STEP NUMBER 4: Avoid snacking by this easy step!

Raise your hand if you have ever gone to the films after your eating window and suddenly wanted some snacks and a gallon of cola? Yep, same here! By choosing the hours once you eat, you'll notice some patterns you didn't concentrate on before. For instance you are the one that just likes to snack while watching TV. So, if you're fasting, for instance, after 7 PM, you've automatically cut hours from your after dinner snacking. So, how could you solve this problem?

Easy as that: getting to bed earlier! You see, building a gentle and regular sleep schedule will assist you minimize food cravings, improve metabolism and can boost your weight loss results.
Another thing: a daily sleep schedule will assist you relieve your stress. High stress causes the body to store fat to guard itself, so by reducing stress, you'll keep the pounds off.
So... GET SOME SLEEP!

STEP NUMBER 5: Don't overindulge in unhealthy food.
You've probably heard it before about fasting: "Eat whatever you want" or "Don't stop eating your favorite foods." This is often true, but most of the time, people take this concept a touch too far. Sure, you'll have a burger once during a while, but having it whenever during your fasting window will ruin all of your results.

While the 16:8 fasting doesn't specify which
foods to eat and avoid, it is vital to specialize in
healthy eating and to limit or avoid junk foods.

 you'll eat what you would like, but you continue
to maintain a diet filled with vegetables, whole
grains and good fats which will keep you full.
confirm you eat enough to form it through your
next fasting window. If you're really hungry
'cause you didn't eat a full meal, you're far more
likely to interrupt your fast!

Listen, guys, just close your kitchen door after
dinner, get more sleep, eat enough to form it
through your next fasting window. and shortly
you'll notice positive results together with your
weight loss and overall health.

Four Beneficial recommendations on the way to Reduce Your Hunger During Intermittent Fasting

Intermittent fasting is an efficient solution to reduce, improve your health, and increase longevity. But there's one minor issue that the majority of you'll experience –hunger. So, here are 4 beneficial recommendations on the way to reduce your hunger during intermittent fasting.

TIP NUMBER 1. Eat Enough Food During Your Eating Window
Even though the key factor of intermittent fasting is the timing of your eating and fasting schedules, what and particularly what proportion you eat is simply as important as once you eat. Remember that fasting isn't a free passport to eat junk food! I like to recommend you stick with high-quality, low-carb, and high-fat meals in

between fasts. specialize in nutrient-dense foods like fruits, veggies, whole grains, nuts, beans, seeds, also as dairy and lean proteins. By the way, there was a study that showed you'll smell bittersweet chocolate to kill your hunger. Crazy, right?

I can't guarantee that you simply won't eat it while smelling it, but you'll provide it a try. Just let my skills work.
Anyways, back to healthy meal choices.
Choosing the proper foods will stabilize your blood sugars, offer you satiety, and make fasting smoother! But remember that consistency is vital to maintaining a successful intermittent fasting routine.

The food quantity and portion size matter even as very much like the standard of food you set into your body. You don't need to obsessively count calories, but you are going to confirm you eat enough to form it through your next fasting window. If you're really hungry because you didn't eat a full meal, you're far more likely to interrupt your fast, which suggests you'll fall out of fat-burning mode.

TIP NUMBER 2: Stay Busy

You'll probably agree that when you're bored, your eat-all-the-food reflex kicks in, even once you aren't really hungry, especially once you start eating ahead of the TV.

Then we've a true problem. Now imagine you're during a fasting state, and you're bored to death. It'll naturally make your fasting harder since you'll have all this point to believe in nothing but food. What I strongly suggest is to form your fasting periods as busy as possible to remain on target. attempt to schedule your activities during your fasting periods.

When you feel hunger pangs, take an extended walk. A brisk walk isn't just a pleasant distraction, but it also maximizes the fat-burning effects when you're fasting. So plow ahead and mix those two for your best results! Another thing you'll distract yourself with is doing household chores, like cleaning or gardening.

I know you're giving a deep sigh immediately because it's going to not sound sort of a fun activity. But believe me: it'll keep you focused on something aside from your hunger and assist you maintain a cleaner, more organized home. But well, if your house is already sparkling clean, you'll also do work-related tasks you've been adjourning, like finishing that report or responding to some emails.

And before going to all those activities before starting your fasting window, put a "CLOSED" check in the fridge. only for your own sake.

TIP NUMBER 3. Build a daily Sleeping Schedule

Sleep is more important to intermittent fasting than you'll possibly imagine. Studies show that sleep is one among the key factors in controlling your appetite because it helps regulate ghrelin, the appetite-stimulating hormone. Lack of sleep results in higher ghrelin levels, which is why you'll feel hungrier once you are sleep deprived.

Building a gentle and regular sleep schedule will assist you balance your hormone levels, minimize food cravings, decrease inflammation in your whole body, and boost your weight loss results.

When you get proper sleep, you'll feel more energized during the day and handle stress easier.

So, there are a couple of effective ways to enhance your sleep quality. Don't erode at least 3 hours before getting to bed, and confirm your bedroom is well ventilated. Also, stick with a daily bedtime schedule and don't attend to sleep too late. I do know you wish to scroll on your phone before bedtime, but attempt to avoid it – read a book instead.

TIP NUMBER 4. Stay Hydrated!
The simplest, easiest, and healthiest method to stave off hunger while fasting is to consume adequate amounts of fluid, especially water.

Thirst can often be confused with a sense of hunger, so keep yourself hydrated. In fact, filling a breast of good, clean water is going to be your favorite weapon to fight hunger.

It also can provide a physical feeling of fullness which can help with true hunger pangs. If you discover it difficult to drink water, especially in the morning, drink sugarless tea or coffee.Similarly to water, a hot beverage won't only offer you a way of fullness but also will occupy the "hand-to-mouth" action, making you feel as if you have eaten.

By the way, a stimulating fact;

One of the studies shows that a little amount of cayenne pepper will reduce your hunger since it causes a shock to your body in a sense that reduces your hunger. So, you'll boost your coffee or tea with a little pinch of cayenne pepper which will help fight your hunger pangs. Just don't overindulge it if you've got issues together with your stomach because it's going to cause a tummy ache!

Alright, so once you start intermittent fasting,
Just steel yourself against hunger, but don't be
scared of it!
Make my suggested ways a habit, and soon,
you'll notice that hunger pangs were just a short-
term inconvenience.

All the required Information you will need to Kickstart a 16:8 Intermittent Fasting Process

You'll be surprised how one thing can make your fasting regime much easier. Okay, so you've chosen the 16:8 method, and for instance your plan is to start out your new regime tomorrow.

Your plan is:
1. Start your fast at 8 PM;
2. Skip breakfast;
3. Have your first meal at 12 PM.

I chose this schedule as an example since most people like it better to skip breakfast and eat from 12 PM to 8 PM. Such a timetable allows them to eat lunch and dinner with friends and family.

Let's undergo your evening before starting your intermittent fasting journey. Have your dinner around 5–7 PM. I'd recommend it to be a low-carb, high-fat meal since it's getting to help satiate you and kickstart you into the advantages of fasting a touch bit sooner.

During your dinner, drink an excellent amount of water because it'll assist you to travel through your fasting hours more easily.

Right before your fasting window, around 7:30 PM, take all of your vitamins and supplements if you're using them.

The reason why you've got to try to do this is often because some supplements, like animal oil or gummies, have calories and can break quickly. Also, you'll eat some yogurt as a dessert before starting your fasting window. At 8 PM, you begin your fast. During your fasting window, you'll only drink water, sugarless, coffee or tea with no added cream or milk.

EXTRA TIPS!

If you want to eat your breakfast, there is no need to push yourself until noon.It's perfectly fine to figure your high thereto. Delay your breakfast for half-hour, then for an hour, and so on. hear your body and do not be hard on yourself. If you discover it too difficult to skip breakfast, be flexible and check out different fasting and eating windows. Each person's lifestyle is different, so do not be afraid to experiment.

Ok, let's head to the morning when you'll fast until 12 PM. Once you awaken, drink a minimum of one glass of water. If you continue to feel hunger pangs, drink another glass or more. Drinking plenty of water throughout the day will keep you full. you'll even have one or two tablespoons of apple vinegar. Taking apple vinegar while fasting may help fight food cravings.

Keep in mind it's extremely acidic, so you'll dilute 1 tablespoon of apple vinegar into 1 cup of water. Then you'll have your black coffee or

tea, again, with no sugar, milk, or cream. Okay, after this lovely morning ritual, you've got a while before breaking your fast.
During this point, attempt to keep yourself as busy as possible so you would not have any temptations to sneak into your fridge. Some people enjoy having their exercise routine within the mornings, so let's mention that a touch.

The first week of fasting could also be difficult since you're adapting to the new regime; you'll feel dizzy and lack some energy.
You might need to go easy on hitting the gym within the beginning
or taking a day off from your workouts just to urge your body to fast. Alright, so your fasting hours have passed and it's already 12 PM. It is time to eat!
While breaking your fast, you do not want to load with a bunch of food. you would like to try to do it strategically.

I recommend starting your eating window with lean protein, like chicken or turkey breast.

Protein helps you reduce by decreasing your energy intake, increasing satiety, and boosting metabolism.

At 1 PM then at 6 PM, have your proper lunch and dinner meal.
You want to make sure you're eating enough during your eating window.
That will ensure you are not hungry the following day during your fasting window. It's super important to incorporate protein, healthy fats, and sophisticated carbs into your meals.

- Figure out your hotel plan

Meal planning doesn't have to be overly restrictive, but your meals have to be strategic and have all the right nutrients. It's super important to trace your water intake. beverages regularly can assist you reduce your calorie intake and can assist you avoid snacking throughout your eating window. Implement exercising into a regime strategically.

- Experiment when is the best time to try to do your workout: during fasting or eating windows.

- Track your weight. If your main goal is to reduce, you would like to trace your weight to stay your motivation up.
- Weigh yourself at an equivalent time a day, and do not weigh yourself quite once each day. Otherwise, it'll become a fanatical habit.

How to get rid of unwanted pounds if all those diets simply don't work?

If you're disgusted by extreme calorie restrictions and unreasonable food limitations, then 16:8 intermittent fasting is strictly what you would like. I'll tell you everything you would like to understand about 16:8 and the way to try to do it right.

First of all, intermittent fasting isn't a diet but an eating approach. The best rule is to limit the time you eat during the day. Different types of intermittent fasting have their eating window once you can consume the food.

There are a couple of ground rules for your eating window

Rule 1: specialize in healthy eating and limit or completely avoid food.

Rule 2: Eat enough nutritious food to form your fasting window easier.

Rule 3: Lower your carb intake. it'll assist you feel less hungry and go longer without eating.

Rule 4: Add enough fat to your everyday meals. Again, this may assist you go longer from one meal to subsequent one.

Rule 5: Add vegetables to each meal since you would like them for magnesium, minerals, and every one the vitamins.

Rule 6: Drink a lot of water!

What you ought to Include In Your Everyday Meals

Ok, I do know it's going to sound overwhelming, so let's go step by step and see what you ought to include in your everyday meals.

1: Protein

Proteins are building blocks of your body. Without them, your body won't be ready to function properly. If you would like to reduce, then you ought to definitely include protein that you simply can see on this list. Such foods will prolong the sensation of satiety and make sure you burn fat without breaking down muscles.

2: Healthy fats

Mono-and polyunsaturated fats are referred to as healthy fats, and that they are an important part of your diet. You'll find healthy fats in fatty fish, like salmon, avocados, nuts, olive or copra oil.

3: Complex carbohydrates

You might have heard that carbs are notorious for causing weight gain. However, whether or not you'll gain weight depends on the sort and quantity of carbs you eat. confirm to settle on foods that are high in fiber and starch but low in sugar. to make it easier for you, here's an inventory of foods that include healthy carbs. you'll also eat apples, bananas, avocados and other fruits,
nuts or vegetables in between your main meals to stay satiated.

4: Water

Proper hydration is extremely important during the day. It promotes skin health, weight loss, and overall wellness. Water also curbs your hunger pangs, cleans out your whole system and effectively removes toxins from your body.
Try drinking 8 glasses of water each day.
Squeezing some lemon or adding one to 2 tablespoons of apple vinegar will add extra benefits.

How Fast are you able to reduce 16:8 Intermittent Fasting?

A person's weight loss pace depends on many factors and varies individually. Technically, the more calories you reduce, the faster you shed pounds. However, that's not always the case. Drastic calorie restriction may cause your body to enter the surviving mode, where you'll stop burning fat and begin burning muscles instead. Health experts recommend losing 1–2 pounds per week. Such a weight loss pace is the safest and therefore the most sustainable.

What Are the Advantages of 16:8 Intermittent fasting?

Intermittent fasting has proven to be an efficient tool in helping people reduce, manage blood sugar levels, and find out how to plan their dinner time properly.

Here are a number of the most health benefits of intermittent fasting:

1: Reduces inflammation
Studies suggest that intermittent fasting could also be effective at helping you reduce inflammation and improve conditions related to inflammation, like arthritis, asthma, Alzheimer's disease, MS and stroke.

2: Lowers the danger of type 2 diabetes
Being overweight and obese are two main risk factors for developing type 2 diabetes. Intermittent fasting could have an impact on

diabetes prevention due to its weight loss effects.
It also can potentially affect other factors.
 A 2014 study showed that intermittent fasting
can lower blood sugar and insulin levels in
people in danger of diabetes.

**3: Promotes the prevention of cardiovascular
diseases**
Studies show that intermittent fasting may
improve your heart health and reduce the danger
of heart diseases.
A 2016 review showed that fasting might reduce
vital signs, pulse, and LDL cholesterol.

4: May reduce the danger of cancer
Numerous animal studies show that intermittent
fasting may reduce the danger of cancer. Such
an impact could also be the aftermath of weight
loss, reduced inflammation, and insulin levels.
Also, a 2019 review in people with cancer states
that fasting reduces the side effects of
chemotherapy and increases its effectiveness.
The review suggests that fasting may deprive

cancer cells of nutrients, making them more vulnerable to the toxins in chemotherapy.

5: Weight loss
One of the most benefits of 16:8 intermittent fasting is weight loss. There are tons of ways during which intermittent fasting can assist you to reduce.
Firstly, fasting lowers insulin levels.This means it becomes easier for your body to use stored fat.

Secondly, eating during a group period can assist you reduce the amount of calories you consume and help boost your metabolism. For instance, one research shows that study participants who practiced intermittent fasting lost three to eight of their weight over 3-24 weeks.

But remember, before beginning to follow any new nutritional plan, it's necessary that you simply consult a dietician or a doctor.

www.ingramcontent.com/pod-product-compliance
Lightning Source LLC
Chambersburg PA
CBHW050756250726
48662CB00005B/2248